The origin of thrombi in the Left Atrium

Alberto Pozo Álvarez

Title:
The origin of thrombi in the Left Atrium

Author:
Alberto Pozo Álvarez

First Edition: July, 2020

Copyright © 2020 Alberto Pozo Álvarez

All rights reserved.

ISBN: 979-8-6675-8575-6

To my loving parents.

Abstract

Approximately 90% of thrombi in atrial fibrillation originate in the left atrium of the heart, specifically in the left atrial appendage. Fluid-dynamic knowledge of the fluid-dynamic behavior of this appendage is still scarce, so there is a need for knowledge in this area. The problem is approached from the point of view of the validation of hemodynamic numerical models and the establishment of adequate boundary conditions.

Table of contents

List of figures — vii

List of tables — ix

Symbols and acronyms — xi

1 Introduction — 1
    1.1 Cardiovascular diseases — 2
    1.2 Computational Fluid Mechanics — 6

2 Thrombus formation in the Left Atrial Appendage — 9
    2.1 Cardiovascular system — 10
        2.1.1 Heart — 10
        2.1.2 Circulation — 13
        2.1.3 Cardiac cycle — 14
    2.2 Left Atrial Appendage — 19
        2.2.1 Left Atrial Appendage Anatomy — 19
        2.2.2 Flow in the Left Atrial Appendage — 22
    2.3 Atrial Fibrillation in the Left Atrial Appendage — 25
    2.4 Cardiac flow visualization techniques — 26

		2.4.1	In vivo techniques..27
		2.4.2	Acquisition of images in the Left Atrial Appendage . 31
	2.5	Percutaneous closure of the Left Atrial Appendage.....................34
		2.5.1	Left Atrial Appendage occlusion 34
		2.5.2	Left Atrial Appendage exclusion....................................37

3 Left Atrial Appendage Computational Models — 39

- 3.1 Blood..40
  - 3.1.1 Density 40
  - 3.1.2 Dynamic viscosity...40
- 3.2 Dimensionless numbers...41
- 3.3 Fluid-mechanical description of the flow in the Left Atrial Appendage 45
  - 3.3.1 Flow pattern..45
  - 3.3.2 Boundary conditions 46
    - 3.3.2.1 Pulmonary veins...47
    - 3.3.2.2 Mitral valve...48
    - 3.3.2.3 Left Atrial Appendage 49
- 3.4 State of the art about the flow in the Left Atrial Appendage . 51

References — 55

List of figures

1.1 Main causes of death in the World in 2016 2
1.2 Stent placement using a catheter 3
1.3 Chaotic electrical signals in patients with atrial fibrillation 5
1.4 Morphological classification of the Left Atrial Appendage 6

2.1 Blood trajectory through the heart chambers 11
2.2 Pressure-Volume changes in the left hemicardium during the cardiac cycle 15
2.3 Section of the heart showing the parts of the left hemicardium   20
2.4 Placement of a Left Atrial Appendage occlusion device 35

3.1 Hagen-Poiseuille velocity profile 41
3.2 Theoretical velocity profile in a cycle for different Womersley numbers 44
3.3 Simplified model of the Left Atrial and Left Atrial Appendage   45
3.4 Estimation of errors in CFD models and in experimental measurements 47
3.5 Flows in a simplified Left Atrial and Left Atrial Appendage model 50

List of tables

2.1 Comparison of image acquisition techniques for LAA evaluation 33

3.1 Pulmonary veins sections obtained with MRI 48

Symbols and acronyms

LAA	Left Atrial Appendage
CFD	Computational Fluid Dynamics
ECG	Electrocardiogram
PIV	Particle Image Velocimetry
Echo-PIV	Echocardiographic Particle Image Velocimetry
Micro-PIV	Microscopic Particle Image Velocimetry
PTV	Particle Tracking Velocimetry
LDV	Laser Doppler Velocimetry
MRI	Magnetic Resonance Imaging
PC-MRI	Phase Contrast Magnetic Resonance Imaging
PC-MRA	Phase Contrast-Magnetic Resonance Angiography
TEE	Transesophageal Echocardiography
TTE	Transthoracic Echocardiography
ICE	Intracardiac Echocardiography
CT	Computed Tomography
MDCT	Multiple Detector Computed Tomography
PET	Positron Emission Tomography
SPECT	Single-Photon Emission Computed Tomography
Re	Reynolds number
Wo	Womersley number
P	Pressure
Q	Flow rate
ρ	Density
μ	Dynamic viscosity
g	Gravitational acceleration

Chapter 1

Introduction

It constitutes a presentation of one of the most common cardiovascular diseases, atrial fibrillation, and its relationship with the Left Atrial Appendage. It is justified the use of Computational Fluid Mechanics (CFD) for the study of cardiovascular diseases.

1.1 Cardiovascular diseases

Heart disease is the first cause of global mortality, as it can be seen in Figure 1.1, whose data have been extracted from the World Health Organization.

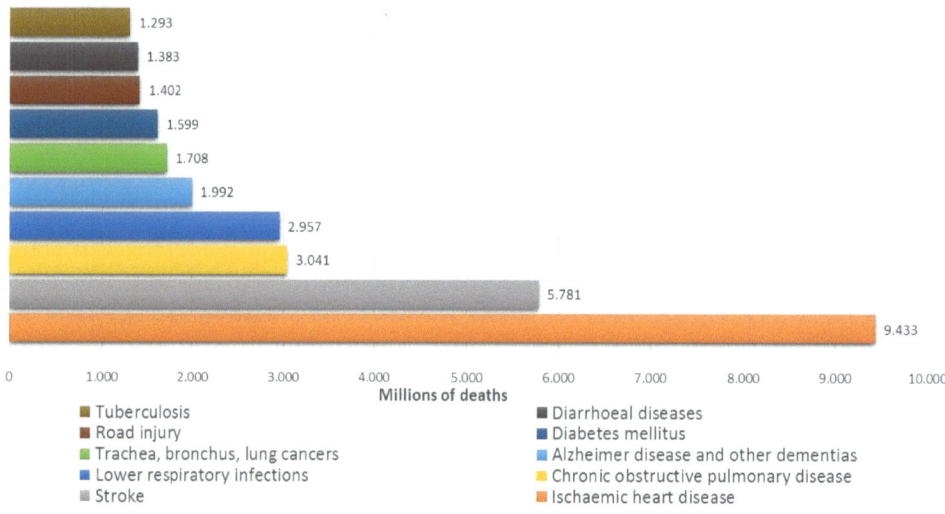

Fig. 1.1 Main causes of death in the World in 2016

Ischemic heart disease is the disease with the highest mortality rate. Within this group the main disease is **atherosclerosis**, consisting of a localized narrowing in arteries caused by accumulation of atheroma plaque, which hinders the blood flow supplied to the heart. This reduction of the section in arteries can cause angina pectoris if it is partial or a heart attack if the obstruction is complete and sudden.

The most widely used method to combat atherosclerotic stenosis is the stent, a tubular metal mesh that is implanted inside the affected artery to recover the cross-sectional area, as it is shown in Figure 1.2.

1.1 Cardiovascular diseases 3

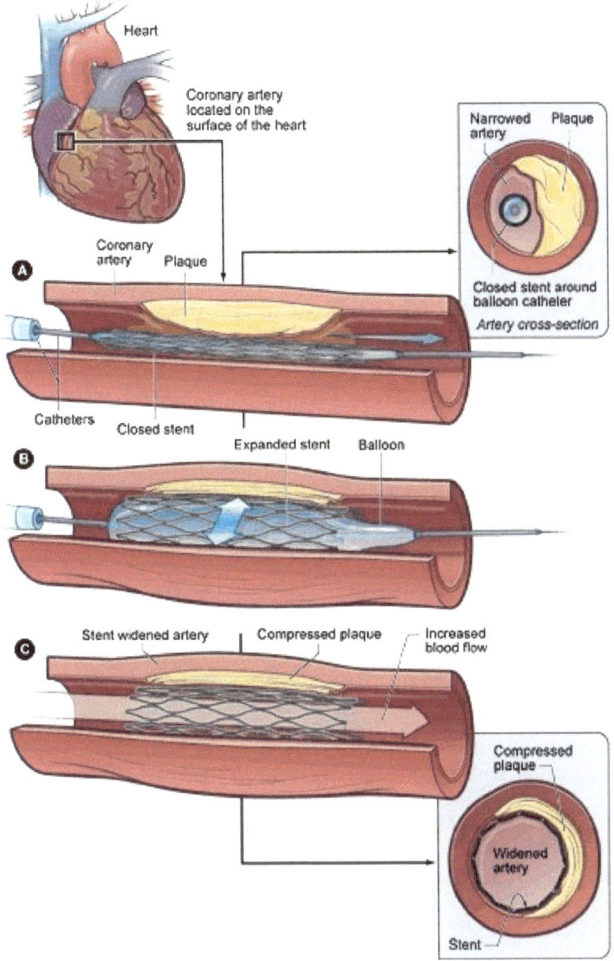

Fig. 1.2 Stent placement using a catheter[1]

---
[1]Creative Commons License (CC0): public domain

On the other hand, the second leading cause of mortality worldwide is cerebrovascular diseases such as hemorrhage, effusion, embolism, thrombosis, cerebral stroke or stroke.

An **embolism** is the obstruction of a blood vessel by a mass which does not dissolve in the blood, an embolus that has been carried away by the blood stream. When the embolism is caused by a thrombus (blood clot) it is called **thrombosis**.

A **stroke** is a sudden attack consisting of an interruption of the blood supply to the brain due to blockage of an artery (ischemic stroke) or because bleeding has occurred (hemorrhagic stroke). **The risk of stroke in patients with atrial fibrillation is 5 to 7 times higher** in comparison with a person who does not suffer from this arrhythmia [58].

In atrial fibrillation, the upper chambers of the heart present chaotic electrical signals causing agitation, especially in the atria. The result is a fast and irregular heartbeat. This disease is one of the most common and important cardiac affections. It is a growing problem in today's society, especially in the oldest, because from 0.4 to 1% of the world population suffers from it, increasing to more than 8% for those over 80 [18].

Particular attention should be paid to the LAA (Left Atrial Appendage) in patients with atrial fibrillation to determine the risk of cardioembolic complications. Approximately 90% of atrial thrombi in nonvalvular atrial fibrillation and 60% of thrombi in patients with rheumatic mitral valve disease (predominantly stenosis) are originated in the LAA [9].

1.1 Cardiovascular diseases

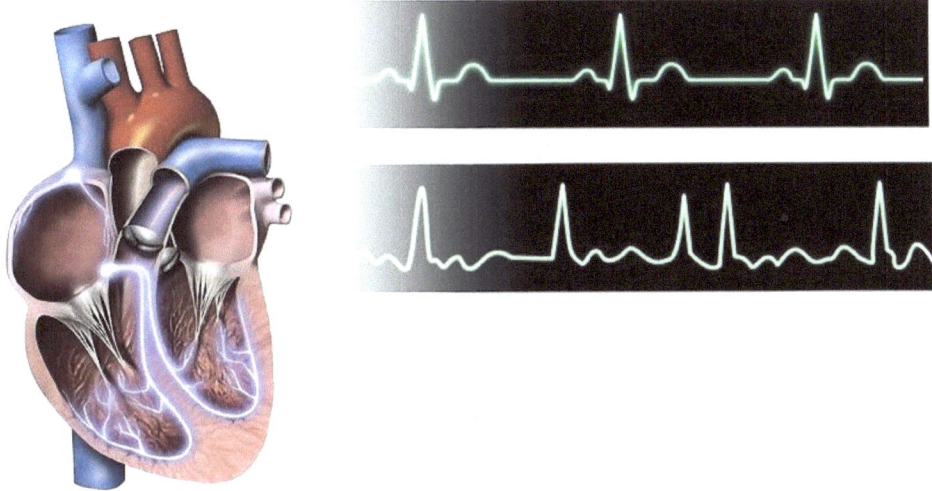

Fig. 1.3 Chaotic electrical signals in patients with atrial fibrillation[2]

The LAA is an appendage located in the Left Atrium of the heart. Atrial fibrillation is thought to produce recirculations of blood in the atrium that may promote thrombus formation in the LAA, where flow conditions are closer to stagnation.

Anselmino et al. [3] showed that there is a correlation between the morphology of the LAA and the risk of stroke in patients with atrial fibrillation. The shape of the LAA is highly variable and at the same time very complex, so it is common to use the morphological classification of Yan et al. [67] with the quantitative limits of Kimura et al. [36]. The four types represented are known as Cactus, ChickenWing, WindSock and CauliFlower, as it can be seen in Figure 1.4.

---

[2]Adapted from: https://commons.wikimedia.org/wiki/File:Atrial_Fibrillation.jpg

6　　　　　　　　　　　　　　　　　　　　　　　　　　Introduction

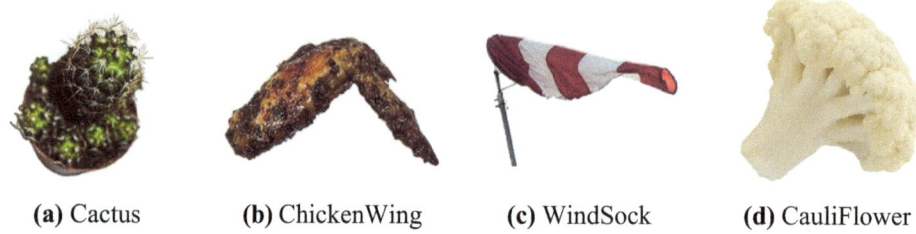

(a) Cactus　　　(b) ChickenWing　　　(c) WindSock　　　(d) CauliFlower

Fig. 1.4 Morphological classification of the Left Atrial Appendage

This Morphological classification of the LAA presented in Figure 1.4 is not so clear since there may be overlapping of the different morphologies when they are viewed from different perspectives, as demonstrated by Beigel et al. [5].

1.2　Computational Fluid Mechanics

In 2000, the Clay Institute of Mathematics located in Cambridge, Massachusetts, announced the seven mathematical problems of the millennium. One of them is the existence and smoothness of the Navier-Stokes Equations, which govern fluid flow in a spatial and temporal domain.

The prediction difficulties of the Navier-Stokes Equations occur at high velocities and small viscosities, when turbulent motion develops.

However, there are some particular solutions to the Navier-Stokes Equations:

- If the non-linear terms are null, we have the Poiseuille flow, the Couette flow or the Stokes law.

- Considering the solutions with non-zero non-linear term, there are some interesting examples such as the Jeffery-Hamel flow, the Von Karman rotary flow or the Taylor-Green vortex, among others.

So there are some mathematicians such as Buckmaster and Vicol working with weak solutions to demonstrate that they are not unique [12].

1.2 Computational Fluid Mechanics

It would mean that for the same initial conditions the same fluid could lead to two different physical states, which makes no physical sense and would indicate that these equations do not describe reality.

Another possibility is that they demonstrate that these solutions are unique, therefore they would have solved the millenium problem.

Pending future work, the only possible mathematical resolution at the moment is numerical. Computational Fluid Mechanics (CFD) is the science in charge of finding a numerical solution of the equations that govern fluid flow in a spatial and temporal domain, the Navier-Stokes equations.

In recent years, it has been demonstrated the usefulness of CFD supported by new imaging or diagnostic techniques for the study of cardiovascular diseases, treatment improvement and prevention [61]. These techniques allow a personalized study of the patient, through the digital twin or virtual patient. These *ad hoc* studies are considered as one of the challenges with the greatest potential impact on cardiovascular biomechanics [31].

One of the main problems that arise within the analysis of virtual patients is the validation of computational codes and their reproducibility [16]. Being numerical models, their results must be validated with experimental tests that confirm their behavior. Of the existing types of validation, two are mainly used: *in vitro* validation [11] and *in vivo* validation [56].

In vivo techniques are those that are carried out directly on the patient's own organism, so in principle they better reflect reality than *in vitro* techniques, which are carried out outside the living organism. As it is not always possible to perform *in vivo* tests, with *in vitro* techniques a much more controlled environment is achieved, which makes them ideal for code validation.

In vitro techniques are based on the use of a fluid with characteristics similar to blood flow that, at the same time, is transparent and with a refractive index similar to that of the model under study in order to carry out the measurement using PIV (Particle Image Velocimetry) technique.

Chapter 2

Thrombus formation in the Left Atrial Appendage

The Left Atrial Appendage is anatomically and functionally described. The study will focus on thrombus formation in the Left Atrial Appendage as a consequence of nonvalvular atrial fibrillation. At the end of the chapter is included a short description of the most used devices to reduce the risk of thrombus formation in the Left Atrial.

2.1 Cardiovascular system

The cardiovascular system is made up of the heart, which acts as an aspirating and impeller pump, and a vascular system composed of arteries, veins and capillaries, thus forming a functional unit which serves the blood, which must be in constant circulation, to irrigate the tissues.

The heart is an organ that has cavities, enclosed in the thoracic cavity, in the center of the chest in a place called mediastinum (mass of tissues located between the sternum and the spinal column). The blood flow in the heart, due to its characteristic velocities and sizes, is highly determined by inertial forces (Re>2500) [62].

2.1.1 Heart

The heart is divided into two halves by a tissue wall, or partition, that runs its entire length. The right half always contains oxygen-poor blood, coming from the superior and inferior vena cava, while the left half of the heart always has oxygen-rich blood. The coming blood from the pulmonary veins will be distributed through the ramifications of the great aorta artery to oxygenate the body's tissues.

Each half of the heart has a superior cavity, the atrium, and another inferior or ventricle, with highly developed muscular walls. There are, therefore, two atria: right and left, and two ventricles: right and left.

2.1 Cardiovascular system

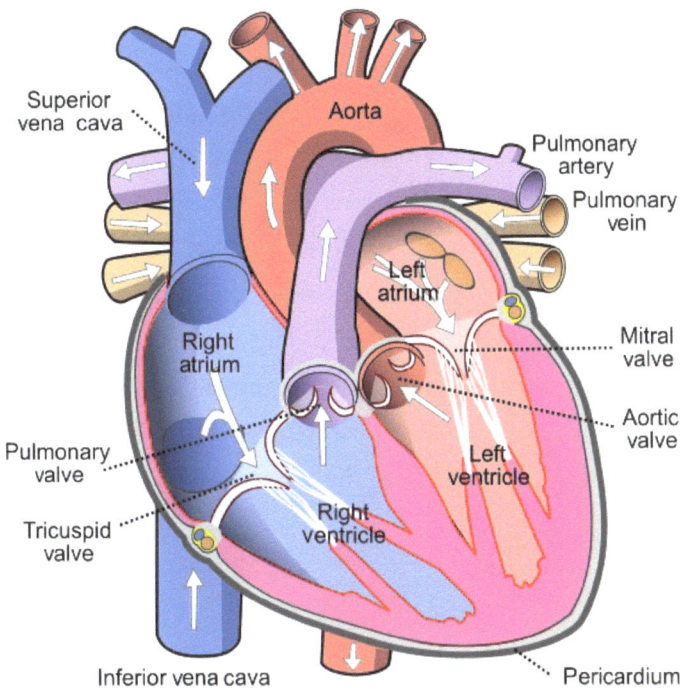

Fig. 2.1 Blood trajectory through the heart chambers[1]

- **Right atrium**

  It is a thin-walled chamber that receives blood from all parts of the body except the lungs. Three large veins empty into it: the superior vena cava, which brings venous blood from the upper body; the inferior cava, which brings venous blood from the lower body, and the coronary sinus, which drains blood from the heart itself. The right atrium pumps deoxygenated (bluish) venous blood into the right ventricle. Blood flows from the right atrium to the right ventricle through the tricuspid valve, consisting mainly of fibrous tissue and so named because it consists of three leaflets or cusps.

---
[1]Creative Commons License (CC0): public domain

- **Right ventricle**

    It is part of the anterior chamber of the heart. Its interior contains a series of ridges, which are formed by the protruding bundles of myocardial fibers, the fleshy trabeculae, some of which contain most of the conduction system and nerve impulses of the heart. The interventricular septum is the division that separates the right ventricle from the left. Blood flows from the right ventricle through the pulmonary semilunar valve to a large artery, the trunk of the pulmonary artery, which is divided into the right and left pulmonary arteries. This chamber must be powerful in propelling blood through the thousands of capillaries in the lungs and back into the left atrium of the heart.

- **Left atrium**

    It forms a large part of the heart base. It receives the already oxygenated blood, coming from the lungs, through the four pulmonary veins. After being received in this chamber, blood is pumped into the left ventricle through the mitral (or bicuspid) valve, which has only two thicker cusps because the left ventricle is the one with the greatest pumping potential.

- **Left ventricle**

    It is the most muscular camera. Its walls are three times thicker than those of the right ventricle. With its powerful pumping, this chamber pumps blood through the aorta to all parts of the body except the lungs. Blood returns to the heart through the right atrium. Blood passes from the left ventricle through the semilunar aortic valve to the body's largest artery, the ascending aorta. From this, a portion flows to the coronary arteries, which branch off from the aorta and carry blood to the aortic arch and descending aorta.

The mitral and tricuspid valves prevent retrograde blood flow from the ventricles to the atria during systole, and the semilunar valves (aortic and pulmonary valves) prevent retrograde flow from the aortic and pulmonary arteries to the ventricles during diastole. These valves close when a retrograde pressure gradient pushes the blood back, and open when a forward pressure gradient forces the blood in an antegrade direction [29].

2.1.2 Circulation

The term circulation refers to movements in a circle or along a circular path. The circulatory system can be studied divided into two smaller circulatory circuits [29]:

- **Minor or pulmonary circulation**: this circuit carries blood from the heart to the lungs and from these to the heart. More specifically, blood travels from the right ventricle through the pulmonary artery to the lungs, the pulmonary arteries rapidly divide into capillaries surrounding the air sacs (alveoli), to exchange oxygen and carbon dioxide. Gradually, the capillaries gather together taking on the characteristics of veins. The veins unite to form the pulmonary veins, which carry oxygenated blood from the lungs to the left atrium.

- **Major or systemic circulation**: this circuit is the main one of the circulation. It carries oxygenated blood from the heart to all regions of the body except the lungs, and then back to the heart. All systemic arteries empty into the inferior or superior vena cava, which in turn flow into the right atrium.

2.1.3 Cardiac cycle

Cardiac events that occur from the beginning of one heart beat to the beginning of the next are called the cardiac cycle. Due to the arrangement of the conduction system there is a delay of more than 0.1 s in the passage of the cardiac impulse from the atria to the ventricles. Blood normally flows continuously from the large veins into the atria, where approximately 80% of the blood flows directly into the ventricles, even before the atria contract. Thereafter, atrial contraction usually results in an additional 20% filling of the ventricles. Thus, the atria act as priming pumps for the ventricles, and the ventricles in turn provide the primary source of power to propel blood through the vascular system [29].

The cardiac cycle is composed of a relaxation period called diastole, followed by a contraction period called systole, as it can be seen in Figure 2.2. The cardiac cycle period is the inverse value of the heart rate. For a heart rate of 75 beats per minute the duration of the cardiac cycle is 0.8 s. The top three curves in Figure 2.2 correspond to pressure changes in the aorta, left ventricle, and left atrium, respectively. Although the atrial pressure remains more or less constant, three small increases in pressure are observed (a, c and v) [29]. The fourth curve represents changes in left ventricular volume, and the fifth represents the electrocardiogram (ECG).

2.1 Cardiovascular system

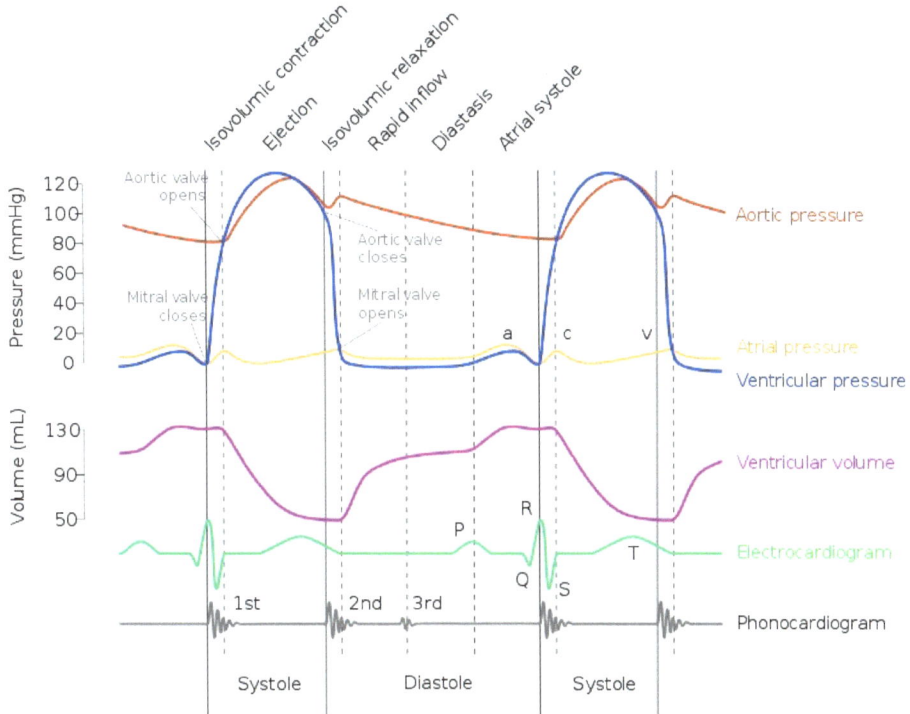

Fig. 2.2 Pressure-Volume changes in the left hemicardium during the cardiac cycle [2]

Seven phases of the cardiac cycle can be distinguished, explained below for the left heart hemicardium. The same events occur in the right hemicardium, with the difference that the pressure in the left hemicardium is significantly higher [17].

---
[2]Adapted from: https://en.wikipedia.org/wiki/File:Wiggers_Diagram_2.svg

- **Phase 1: atrial contraction.** This phase begins with the **P wave** corresponding to the electrocardiogram. This wave is produced by the propagation of depolarization in the atria and has a duration of 50 ms approximately [70]. It corresponds to the last part of ventricular diastole, in which all the chambers are relaxed and the left ventricle is partially filled with blood. There is hardly any flow through the mitral valve at this stage because left atrium and left ventricle pressures are practically the same. When the atrium contracts, the pressure inside it increases, causing additional blood flow to the left ventricle, corresponding to **a wave** in the diagram. Usually the right atrial pressure increases from 4 to 6 mmHg during atrial contraction and the left atrial pressure increases from approximately 7 to 8 mmHg [29]. The pressure in the left atrium exceeds the pressure in the veins, but only small amounts of reverse flow take place. Atrial systole lasts for about 100 ms.

- **Phase 2: isovolumic contraction.** This is the first stage of ventricular systole. Approximately 150 ms after the start of the P wave, **QRS waves** (90 ms of duration) appear as a consequence of electrical depolarization of the ventricles, which initiates contraction of the ventricles and an elevation of ventricular pressure [70]. As the pressure inside the ventricle exceeds the atrial pressure, the mitral valve closes immediately. The ventricle is now a closed chamber. For a short period of time the pressure continues to build rapidly while valves are closed. During this phase there are no changes in volume, that is why it is said to be isovolumetric. The rapid increase in left ventricular pressure causes the mitral valve to buckle into the left atrium, this can be seen in a small spike in the atrial pressure curve, the **c wave**.

2.1 Cardiovascular system

- **Phase 3: rapid ejection.** Once the pressure in the left ventricle exceeds the pressure in the aorta (approximately 80 mmHg), the aortic valve opens and a rapid ejection of blood into the aorta begins. The ventricular muscles begin to shorten, and the volume of the ventricle decreases. The pressure gradient between the aorta and the left ventricle is very small due to the large opening of the aortic valve (low resistance). As a result of contraction and shortening of the left ventricle, the mitral annulus descends and the left atrium expands slightly with a pressure drop occurring in the left atrium. Venous blood continues to pass into the left atrium, and the atrial pressure increases again.

- **Phase 4: reduced ejection. T wave** is observed in the electrocardiogram, representing the repolarization of the ventricles, when the fibers of the ventricular muscle begin to relax. This wave lasts approximately 50 ms and occurs 250 ms after the QRS complex ends [70]. The pressure in the left ventricle is reduced and the period of reduced ejection begins. The pressure in the left ventricle gradually decreases and falls slightly below the pressure in the aorta, which is also decreasing. In- stead, blood continues to leak from the left ventricle due to inertia. At the end of systole, the pressure in the left ventricle drops faster and reverse blood flow to the left ventricle appears. Blood flows to the cusps of the aortic valve, which closes abruptly. Passive filling of the atrium continues during this period until the end of the fifth phase.

  For a normal person at rest, ventricular systole (phases 2, 3 and 4) usually lasts about 270 ms [37].

- **Phase 5: Isovolumic relaxation.** After the aortic valve closes, the ventricle continues to relax and the pressure drops dramatically. The left ventricle volume remains constant because all the valves are closed. This is the beginning of ventricular diastole. The pressure in the atrium now reaches its maximum, as can be seen at the peak of the **v wave**.

- **Phase 6: rapid filling.** When the pressure in the left ventricle falls below the pressure in the left atrium, the mitral valve opens rapidly. The blood accumulated in the atrium during systole now flows into the left ventricle. Pressure in the left ventricle and left atrium continues to drop, that of the atrium because it is emptying into the ventricle and that of the ventricle because it is still under relaxation. Ongoing relaxation of the left ventricle creates additional suction of blood from the left atrium. The volume in the left atrium decreases while the left ventricle is expanding.

- **Phase 7: reduced filling.** As the left ventricle continues to fill and expand, the pressure in the left ventricle begins to increase again. This reduces the pressure gradient between the two chambers and the filling slows down. During this period the pulmonary veins fill the left atrium and restore a positive atrioventricular pressure gradient.

Ventricular diastole comprises phases 5, 6, 7 and 1 and lasts approximately 530 ms for a person with a heart rate of 75 beats per minute.

2.2 Left Atrial Appendage

There are two appendages in the heart, located in each atrium, one in the right hemicardium and the other in the left hemicardium, which is the one that will be the object of study in this work.

2.2.1 Left Atrial Appendage Anatomy

The Left Atrial Appendage (LAA) is an additional, finger-shaped cavity that originates from the wall of the Left Atrium. The junction with the left atrium is defined by a narrow orifice called **ostium** that gives access to this cavity. There is a wide variety of sizes and shapes for this appendage, discovered thanks to TEE (Transesophageal Echocardiography). Its relationship with the adjacent cardiac and extracardiac structures can be highly relevant when an intervention is required [5]. The LAA derives from the left wall of the primary atrium, but has different physiological characteristics than the Left Atrium. It is found in the confines of the pericardium in close relationship with the free wall of the left ventricle, hence its emptying and filling is significantly affected by the function of the left ventricle [2].

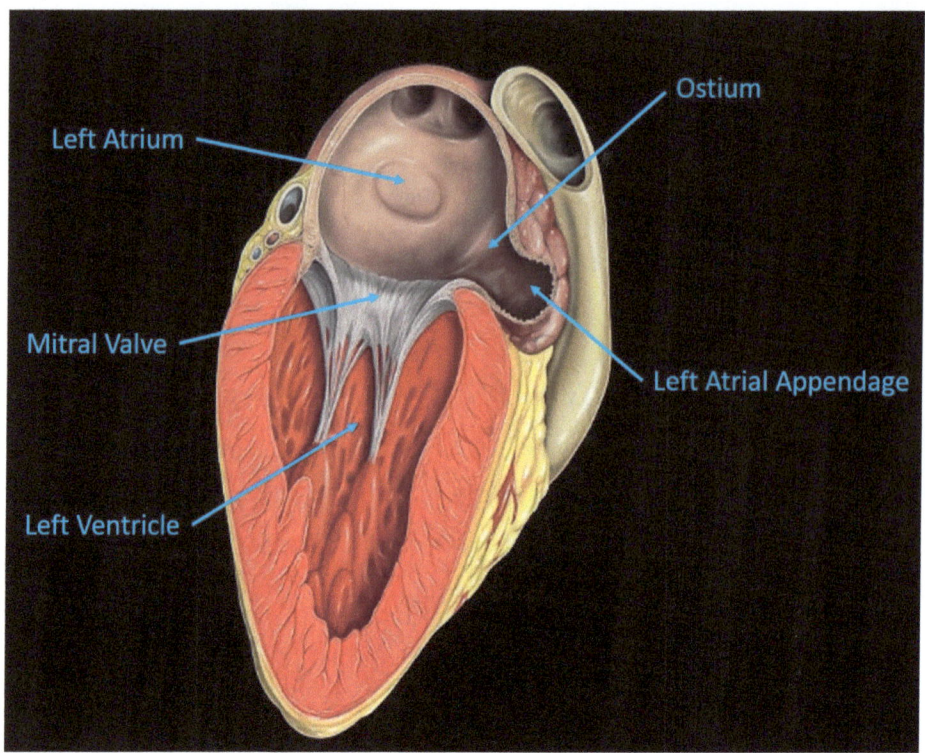

Fig. 2.3 Section of the heart showing the parts of the left hemicardium [3]

The external appearance of the LAA is that of a slightly flattened tubular structure with battlements, often with one or more folds and ending in a pointed tip, which is usually directed laterally and towards the rear. Due to its slightly flattened shape, the lower surface is generally on the Left Ventricle and the upper surface is below the fibrous pericardium. Internally, the orifice of the appendage (ostium) is usually oval, while the round, triangular, and raindrop shapes are less common [67].

The left lateral flange separates the Left Pulmonary Vein orifices from Ostium, but the precise relationship between the level of the orifice and its distance from the venous orifices varies [42].

---

[3]Adapted from: https://commons.wikimedia.org/wiki/File:Heart_left_atrial_appendage_tee_view.jpg

2.2 Left Atrial Appendage

One of the first studies of the LAA anatomy was carried out by Ernst et al. [21] studying its morphology using synthetic resin molds made at autopsy. In 198 of the cases they had an antemortem ECG (143 with sinus rhythm and 55 with atrial fibrillation). The results offered large variations in sizes:

- The volume of the molds was between 0.7 and 19.2 mL.

- The diameter of the Ostium varied from 10 to 40 mm.

- The length of the LAA ranged from 16 to 51 mm.

Samples from patients who had suffered from atrial fibrillation were more voluminous, with larger orifices and less ramifications than those of sinus rhythm. In a large postmortem study of hearts by Veinot et al. [64] lobes were defined as protuberances of the main body with the tail portion, while the curves in the tail do not constitute more lobes. He found that 2 lobes were the most common (54%), followed by 3 lobes (23%), 1 lobe (20%) and 4 lobes (3%). No differences were found in the morphology of the LAA related to the age or sex of the person. A higher number of lobes has been associated with the presence of thrombi, regardless of clinical risk and blood stasis [68]. Di Biase et al. [8] used MDCT (Multidetector Computed Tomography) and MRI (Magnetic Resonance Imaging) to classify the shapes of LAA in patients with chronic atrial fibrillation into 4 morphological types: ChickenWing, the most common with 48%, Cactus (30%), WindSock (19%) and CauliFlower (3%).

- **ChickenWing**: it has a dominant lobe that shows an angulation in its proximal or middle portion, returning towards the origin (Ostium). This type of LAA may have secondary lobes with different orientation from the main lobe.

- **Cactus**: it is characterized by a dominant central lobe with secondary lobes extending from the central lobe in upper and lower directions. Such variations are related to the number, location, and orientation of the secondary lobes.

- **Windsock**: a dominant lobe of sufficient length constitutes the primary structure. Variations arise with the location and number of secondary or even tertiary lobes emerging from the dominant lobe in the inferior direction.

- **Cauliflower**: its main characteristic is that it has a limited total length with more complex internal characteristics. Variations of this type show a usually irregular morphology of the Ostium (oval vs. round), a variable number of lobes present, the absence of a dominant lobe, and the proximity of internal separations or ridges near the Ostium.

According to the study carried out by Di Biase et al. [8] the LAA morphology **Cauliflower** presents the highest thromboembolic risk.

However, as demonstrated by Beigel et al. [5] this classification is not as clear as one might think because there may be overlapping of the different morphologies when they are viewed from different angles.

2.2.2 Flow in the Left Atrial Appendage

The LAA acts as a buffer chamber during ventricular systole and during periods of high pressure in the Left Atrium [2].

It shows a contraction pattern different from the rest of the Left Atrium because it contracts more. Blood flow within the LAA has been studied with TEE, which provides good views of the appendix and its orifice. The flow of LAA measured by Doppler in patients with sinus rhythm was described as biphasic [27]. With the onset of diastole, the left ventricle relaxes and the LAA empties, causing flow out through the mitral valve. Coincident with atrial systole, there is additional forward flow due to LAA contraction. With ventricular systole (the left ventricle contracts), a reentrant flow is initiated in LAA, thanks to its elasticity [2].

2.2 Left Atrial Appendage

Fyrenius et al. [25] performed a study of the flow inside the heart on 11 healthy patients, using MRI. From the velocity fields they obtained paths, streamlines and transit times.

They observed that the entry of blood from the right pulmonary veins is done smoothly through the atrial wall, while the left veins do a more sudden entry redirecting towards the mitral valve.

Two temporal vortices were identified in all subjects in the left atrium during systole and toward mid-diastole. The rotation axis of both vortices is crescent-shaped and parallel to the plane of the mitral annulus.

Flow from the left pulmonary vein contributes most of the volume incorporated into the atrial vortices, both in systole and in mid-diastole. Instead, the right pulmonary venous flow is restricted between the periphery of the vortex and the atrial wall.

The following stages are distinguished in terms of the development of the vortices in the left atrium:

- **Ventricular systole**. Vortical flow in the left atrium begins to develop just before ventricular systole, and increases in magnitude during systole. The diameters of the vortices towards the end of the systole are between 2.5 and 3.5 cm. The vortex disappears at the beginning of diastole. The total duration of the systolic vortex is 280 ms, regardless of heart rate.

- **Early diastole**. Blood from the four pulmonary veins passes directly into the left atrium and passes through the mitral valve during rapid ventricular emptying during diastole.

- **Diastole**. A second vortex in the left atrium develops toward the middle of diastole. Vortical flow appears following the incoming flow peak at the beginning of diastole and its diameter reaches its maximum value towards the middle of diastole, with values between 3.3 and 2.2 cm.

From inception to disappearance with atrial contraction, the vortex duration was 256 ms, although it was highly dependent on heart rate.

- **Atrial contraction**. The vortex of half of the diastole is extinguished with atrial contraction and retraction of the mitral annulus. Streamlines showed reverse flow of atrial blood to the pulmonary veins and forward flow through the mitral valve.

They identified inflow from the LAA during atrial contraction in 9 of the 11 subjects. Streamlines showed a small area of flow propulsion from the appendage to the left atrium, with recirculation to the LAA during subsequent relaxation.

The vortices that appear in systole and towards the middle of diastole are the result of the disparate interaction of the incoming flow of the right and left pulmonary veins with the walls of the atrium and with the other part of the flow during the phases of the cardiac cycle, when the blood output from the atrium decreases or stops. The residual volume present in the atrium at the beginning of these stages is carried away by the incoming flow and incorporated into the vortex, thus avoiding a complete deceleration. Flow from the right pulmonary veins follows the vortex at its periphery, restricted between the vortex and the atrial wall. As a result, instead of expanding to the width of the left atrium and decelerating proportionally, the right inflow is limited to a narrow passage that preserves its velocity and direction toward the mitral valve. At the same time, the velocities of the incoming right flow at the periphery of the vortex to the left could increase its duration. This different behavior of the flow from the right and left pulmonary veins is present during systole, when the mitral valve is closed, and during half of diastole, when a relative direct passage of the incoming flow from the right pulmonary veins coexists with a recirculation just above a partially closed mitral valve [25].

Besides acting as flywheels accumulating kinetic energy vortexes prevent the appearance of stasis and hence the blood clotting inside the left atrium.

2.3 Atrial fibrillation in the Left Atrial Appendage

In atrial fibrillation, the upper chambers of the heart present chaotic electrical signals causing agitation, especially in the atria. The result is a fast and irregular heartbeat. This disease is one of the most common and important cardiac affections and is a growing problem in today's society, especially in the elderly, since 0.4 to 1% of the world population suffers from it, increasing to more than 8 % for those over 80 [5].

Particular attention should be paid to the LAA in patients with atrial fibrillation to determine the risk of cardioembolic complications. Approximately 90% of atrial thrombi in nonvalvular atrial fibrillation and 60% of thrombi in patients with rheumatic mitral valve disease (predominantly stenosis) are originated in the LAA [9].

In a study of Di Biase et al. [7] the LAA appears to be responsible for cardiac arrhythmias in 27% of patients.

Thrombus formation is more likely to occur within the LAA when reduced contractility occurs and stasis occurs in its cavity. During atrial fibrillation, a decrease in contractility occurs, causing the velocities within it to decrease and the LAA to dilate, causing it to function as a static bag that predisposes to stagnation and thrombosis [49].

In patients without cardiac abnormalities, emptying speeds in the LAA range from 50 to 80 cm/s and filling rates from 46 to 60 cm/s. In patients with elevated pressure in the left atrium the velocities are lower, as in patients with atrial fibrillation. In the latter, the flow pattern is more variable [60].

Patients with significant left ventricular dysfunction and elevated pressures in left ventricular diastole may also be at risk for thrombus formation in LAA in absence of atrial fibrillation [65]. Speeds below 20 cm/s are usually associated with a risk of thrombus development in the LAA and which may cause a cerebral embolism if they are subsequently transmitted to the brain through the circulatory system [44].

Consequently, the risk of thrombus formation in LAA appears to be related to altered LAA function, reduced contraction capacity, and elevated filling pressures, regardless of cause. LAA thrombi are present in up to 14% of patients with acute atrial fibrillation [59].

2.4 Cardiac flow visualization techniques

The following classification regarding cardiac flow measurement techniques can be established:

- *In vivo* **techniques.** Those that are carried out directly on the patient's organism, that is why they reflect best the reality a priori. They do not require direct visual access to the study area.

- *In vitro* **techniques.** They are performed outside the living organism. As it is not always possible to perform *in vivo* tests, with the *in vitro* techniques a much more controlled environment is achieved, which makes them ideal for the validation of numerical codes. They require direct visual access to the study region.

- *In silico* **techniques.** Refers to computational studies performed using numerical CFD simulation. These numerical models need an *in vivo* or *in vitro* validation.

2.4 Cardiac flow visualization techniques

2.4.1 In vivo techniques

There are several *in vivo* techniques based on clinical images that make it possible to characterize the functioning of the heart:

- **Echocardiography**, based on the use of ultrasound. There are different types:

    - **TTE (Transthoracic echocardiography)**. It is a non-invasive technique and constitutes the most common type of echocardiogram. The ultrasonic transducer is placed on the chest wall and varying its position and orientation, images of different planes of the heart can be obtained. This technique allows the reconstruction of 2D and 3D images.

    - **TEE (Transesophageal Echocardiography)**. It is an invasive technique consisting of the introduction of an ultrasonic transducer through the patient's esophagus. This technique is used more frequently when transthoracic images are not optimal and greater precision is needed for evaluation, such as in case of heart valves. It allows obtaining 2D and 3D images.

    - **ICE (Intracardiac Echocardiography)**. Provides high-resolution images from inside the heart with the introduction of a venous catheter.

- **Doppler echocardiography**. It is a variety of traditional echocardiography in which, taking advantage of the Doppler effect, it is possible to determine if the flow is directed towards or away from the transducer. The velocity component of such flow can only be determined along the transducer direction by Equation 2.1.

$$v = \frac{(f_e - f_r) \cdot c}{2 f_e \cdot \cos\theta} \qquad (2.1)$$

In Equation 2.1 v is the velocity to be estimated, f_e the emission frequency, f_r the reception frequency, θ the angle between the ultrasound beam and the object under study and c is the velocity of sound transmission in the tissues. The angle θ must be as close to 0 (aligned ultrasound beam and study object) because the cosine would be 1 and the velocity measurement would be exact.

There are three types of Doppler applied to the study of blood flow [54]:

- **Pulsed Doppler**. The transducer emits an ultrasound pulse and after a certain time, depending on the depth of the measurement point, receives it. In this way, the flow velocity at the point on the line where the sample volume is located is known. Its main limitation is the inability to measure high velocities (>1 m/s).

- **Continuous Doppler**. The transducer emits and receives simultaneously, so that it does not have a repetition pulse rate limitation and therefore can register high velocities (even higher than 6 m/s). It registers the velocities in the entire ultrasound beam and not in a specific point, unlike Pulsed Doppler. The spectrum representation does not allow to differentiate near and far fluxes.

2.4 Cardiac flow visualization techniques

- **Color Doppler**. This is a variant of Pulsed Doppler that represents a color-coded average velocity map, superimposed on the two-dimensional image of the cardiac anatomy. This information is obtained in the same way as with Pulsed Doppler, simultaneously interrogating multiple sample volumes sequentially on a selected surface called color box, coded with a different color depending on the direction of the detected movement.

    Color Doppler enables the rapid display of large amounts of information of hemodynamic interest. However, it does not represent the maximum velocity but the average velocity. Also, *Aliasing* can appear easily as the Nyquist limit can be reached for flows with speeds not excessively high (0.6 m/s) [53].

- **Echo-PIV (Echocardiographic Particle Image Velocimetry)**. Technique based on cross-correlation of particle image fields acquired by ultrasound. It is derived from optical PIV, which is a usually two-dimensional *in vitro* technique but can allow 3D visualization of the flow by combining measurements in multiple planes, so it does not have the limitations of Doppler. Multiphase bubbles of a gas with a hydrophilic envelope are used as contrast agents. The size of these bubbles must coincide with that of the red blood cells to avoid blockage of the pulmonary capillaries when administered intravenously. Inside the arteries and the heart, these bubbles create aggregates that generate great dispersion when under an ultrasound field. Echo-PIV uses these aggregates as tracer particles [6].

    A limitation of this technique is related to the complex interaction of ultrasound with bubble aggregates. This causes the tracers to disappear from the image plane, not only because of out-of-plane movements, but also because ultrasound energy can implode the bubbles, increasing noise. In addition, it only allows speeds below 0.4 m/s to be measured because it does not have sufficient precision for higher velocities [55].

- **MDCT (Multidetector Computed Tomography)**. This technique is called Computed Tomography (CT) because it is possible to obtain images of tomographic sections reconstructed in non-transverse planes. Instead of obtaining a projection image, like conventional radiography, CT obtains multiple images making the X-ray source and radiation detectors rotate movements around the body. The final representation of the tomographic image is obtained capturing the signals by the detectors and post-processing them using reconstruction algorithms. With this technique, a level of detail less than a millimeter can be obtained for the anatomy over time, making it ideal for cardiac geometry studies [41].

- **MRI (Magnetic Resonance Imaging)**. It is a non-invasive technique thanks to which a detailed three-dimensional reconstruction of the anatomy can be performed obtaining images in different measurement planes. Unlike what happens with CT (Axial Computed Tomography) does not use ionizing radiation. It uses magnets that produce a powerful magnetic field that forces the hydrogen atoms in the body to align with that field. When a radio frequency current is pulsed, protons are stimulated and perform an out-of-equilibrium precession motion. When that radio frequency field is turned off, the sensors detect the energy released while the protons are realigning with the magnetic field as well as the time until that realignment.

  PC-MRI (Phase Contrast—Magnetic Resonance Imaging) is a specific type of MRI that measures the velocity of blood flow in any arbitrary direction of the magnetic field gradient, and is based on the principle that the PC-MRI offset is proportional to the speed of the moving proton. Modern PC-MRI is typically time-resolved and provides a flow velocity vector distribution in all three directions of space (usually anterior-posterior, left-right, and superior-inferior). For this reason, it is also known as 3D cine PC-MRI or 4D flow MRI[33].

2.4 Cardiac flow visualization techniques

2.4.2 Acquisition of images in the Left Atrial Appendage

Due to the complex anatomical characteristics of thrombi, its detection in the LAA, a small area with a multilobed anatomy, can cause difficulties.

- **Transesophageal Echocardiography (2D and 3D TEE).** Imaging with 3D TEE is a relatively recent development that improves the anatomical evaluation of LAA. Although TEE 2D provides higher resolution images, TEE 3D allows a more complete evaluation of LAA overcoming some of the limitations associated with 2D images, such as inadequate image planes. In addition, TEE 3D provides better separation and differentiation between adjacent structures, along with a more complete and comprehensive evaluation of LAA, its complex morphology, and the surrounding structures [48]. The sensitivity of the 3D TEE to detect thrombi in the LAA is still limited, although with recent advances in the development of percutaneous devices for closure of the LAA, 3D TEE has gained in importance in guiding the device to the LAA [43].

- **Intracardiac Echocardiography (ICE).** It can provide multiple views and detailed images of the LAA to diagnose the presence of thrombi [20]. Although ICE is less sensitive compared to TEE for thrombus detection, it can serve as a complementary method, especially when TEE results warrant further evaluation. However, because ICE is an invasive procedure, its use is limited in daily practice and is primarily reserved for catheterization during planned cardiac procedures.

- **Doppler.** Doppler echocardiography is used to assess the risk of thromboembolism in the LAA estimating velocity because TEE has limited sensitivity identifying small thrombi within the lateral lobes, even with three-dimensional images [5].

- **Comparison with other imaging techniques:** Although TEE is the most widely used method for evaluation of the LAA, MDCT and MRI are emerging as valuable modalities for imaging and evaluation of the anatomy and functionality of the LAA. Table 2.1 summarizes the main strengths and limitations of each imaging modality. MDCT and MRI are likely to play an increasingly important role in the preoperative and postoperative assessment of LAA when its image resolution is improved to allow accurate determination of thrombus [5].

MRI is a non-invasive alternative for those cases where TEE is not possible, such as in patients with esophageal pathologies or who have had a failed probe insertion during TEE. However, this modality has been evaluated in a limited number of studies. MRI can accurately visualize the size and function of the LAA and has the potential to detect thrombi in patients with atrial fibrillation [13]. The sensitivity of MRI identifying the presence of thrombi in the LAA is somewhat lower than with MDCT. Although MRI has many advantages over MDCT and TEE, such as the absence of exposure to iodine contrast and radiation without the need of the introduction of a probe, it still has many limitations for its extended use: low temporal resolution (more than 30 ms), prolonged exploration time, respiratory dependency and impossibility of application in patients with implanted cardiac devices [6]. Furthermore, its spatial resolution, usually greater than 1mm voxel, is not sufficient to address a small region such as the LAA [45].

TTE and TEE can be used to measure the velocity of blood flow in both the left atrium and left atrial appendage, but both techniques only provide averaged information of the velocity module and its direction in the measurement volume, without giving detailed 3D information of local flow conditions [19].

2.4 Cardiac flow visualization techniques

Table 2.1 Comparison of image acquisition techniques for LAA evaluation [5]

	TEE	MDCT	MRI
Sensitivity/specificity for thrombi detection	92%-100%/ 98%-99%	96% / 92%	67% / 44%
Spatial resolution	0.2-0.5 mm	0.4 mm	1-2 mm
Temporal resolution	20-30 ms	70-105 ms	30-50 ms
3D Volume Rendering	With 3D	Yes	Yes
Contrast required	No*	Yes	No*
Ionizing radiation	No	Yes	No
Availability	Wide	Limited	Limited
Type of technique	Invasive	Non-invasive	Non-invasive
Real-time evaluation	Yes	No	No
Special considerations		Dynamic evaluation of LAA	Incompatible with pacemakers

*Contrast can be used to improve visualization of thrombi in doubtful cases

2.5 Percutaneous closure of the Left Atrial Appendage

In people with atrial fibrillation over 65 years, the usual treatment to reduce the risk of thrombosis is oral anticoagulants [47].

Although the incidence of thromboembolism can be dramatically reduced by this treatment, a TEE study found that 1.6% of patients treated with anticoagulants for 1 month had echocardiographic evidence of a thrombus in the LAA [57]. Furthermore, for certain patients the use of anticoagulants may be contraindicated due to the high risk of bleeding, therefore alternative forms of treatment for thromboembolism prophylaxis are needed in these patients [2]. One of them, which is currently in evolution, is the LAA closure device, which serves to prevent the occurrence of embolic events in patients with nonvalvular atrial fibrillation [26]. There are two strategies for percutaneous closure of the LAA: occlusion and exclusion.

2.5.1 Left Atrial Appendage occlusion

The occlusion consists of the placement of an intravascular device in the LAA percutaneously, through a venous access. The two most commonly used devices for the LAA occlusion are the Watchman device (Boston Scientific Corp., Natick, Massachusetts) and the Amplatzer-Amulet (St. Jude Medical, Inc., St. Paul, Minnesota) [4]. Both are implanted transseptally through the femoral vein, are highly flexible and have a stabilizer guide system that anchors to the wall of the LAA and thus prevents embolization.

2.5 Percutaneous closure of the Left Atrial Appendage

- The **Watchman** device is a kind of plug formed by a nitinol network or structure and is covered with a 160 micron polyethylene terephthalate (PET) membrane designed to prevent thrombus leakage and favor endothelialization. It has 10 active fixation anchors to hold the tissue and achieve the necessary stability to remain fixed to the LAA. As there is no disc, it cannot interfere with the pulmonary veins or the mitral valve. The Watchman system is implanted 10 mm from the Ostium of the LAA and therefore does not cover it.

- The **Amplatzer-Amulet** device is made of highly flexible nitinol mesh. The design is circular, it is made up of a stopper or lobe and a disc, joined by a waist that acts as a very flexible joint, which allows it to adapt and accommodate itself when released. The plug or lobe attaches to the inner wall of the LAA and the hooks or lobe stabilization guides help its internal fixation. The disc is designed to cover the entrance orifice of the LAA and must be embedded in it, pulled by the plug. With this system, the lobe is implanted 10 mm deep from the Ostium and the disc completely covers the Ostium of the LAA [22].

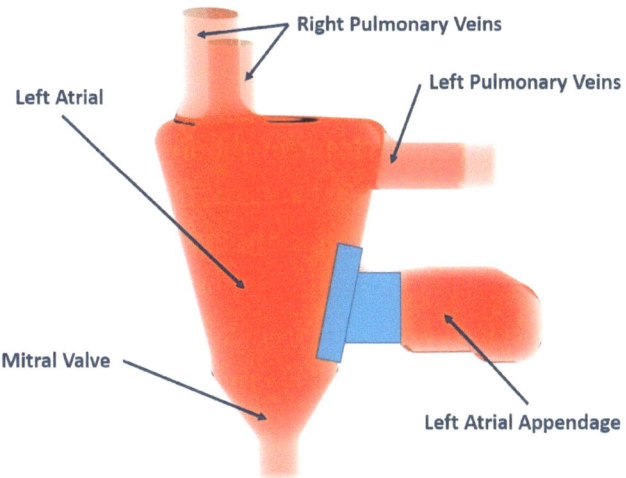

Fig. 2.4 Placement of a Left Atrial Appendage occlusion device

In the procedure carried out for the occlusion of the LAA, the catheter is introduced through the femoral vein to access the inferior vena cava and the interatrial septum. The procedure to be followed during the intervention is as it follows [22]:

1. **Transseptal puncture.** It is recommended to puncture in the inferior and posterior areas of the oval fossa. The positioning of the needle, the transseptal puncture and the canalization of the LAA must be controlled by TEE.

2. **Probing of the left atrium and Left Atrial Appendage.** Once the left atrium has been accessed, a guide is advanced to the LAA. Full visualization of intracardiac catheters and devices is extremely important to avoid complications because any sudden movement can cause perforation or plugging due to fragility of the LAA wall.

3. **Measurement of the Left Atrial Appendage and choice of device.** It is neccesary to know the dimensions of the Ostium as well as the length and depth of the appendage to plan the introduction of the LAA occlusion device. For this, image acquisition techniques are used, such as TEE and MDCT, which allow determining the suitability for the implantation of said device [49].

4. **Deployment, positioning and release of the device.** Once the lobe has been deployed in the landing area, the disc is released, which should have a concave-convex morphology, ideally embedded in the entrance of the LAA. Before releasing the device, it must be checked that it is properly seated and occlusive, with no residual flow in the appendage. Furthermore, it should not affect neighboring structures such as the mitral valve or the circumflex artery.

However, according to a study by Kanderian et al. [35], 11% of the patients in whom the closure of the LAA has been successfully carried out suffer strokes again. Thrombus formation would take place in the left atrium but upon closure of the LAA if the device has not been properly selected, so the exclusion of the LAA could avoid this risk.

2.5.2 Left Atrial Appendage exclusion

The exclusion of the LAA from circulation is achieved applying an external ligation. Currently, there is only one device for LAA exclusion: the LARIAT latch device (SentreHEART Inc., Redwood City, California), which uses a ligation suture to exclude the LAA [5].

Chapter 3

Left Atrial Appendage Computational Models

A fluid dynamic characterization of the flow in the heart is performed, specifically in the Left Atrium and Left Atrial Appendage. This step is very important to establish adequate boundary conditions in hemodynamic numerical models.

3.1 Blood

3.1.1 Density

Blood is an incompressible fluid due to the large amount of water it has. This means that the density of the blood remains constant with pressure changes, although it may vary from person to person depending on their metabolism. It is usually considered a constant value of 1055 kg/m^3 [66].

3.1.2 Dynamic viscosity

Blood is a non-Newtonian fluid. Despite the fact that plasma behaves like a Newtonian fluid, the presence of red blood cells (hematocrit), which account for up to 99% of the particles present in the blood, do the viscosity variable. This is modified depending on the dimensions of the tube and the type of flow. When the blood velocity increases, the viscosity decreases.

The viscosity of the blood depends drastically on the hematocrit, increasing its value when the hematocrit percentage is higher. For normal physiological blood levels of around 40% hematocrit percentage, a mean blood viscosity value of 3.5 centipoise (0.0035 Pa·s) is considered at the temperature of 38°C [66]. Although its rheological behavior is fundamentally different, blood is usually modeled as a Newtonian fluid.

3.2 Dimensionless numbers

The Reynolds number is used to determine if a flow is laminar or turbulent. For a straight and rigid circular section duct, the Reynolds number from which the flow is considered turbulent is 2300.

$$Re = \frac{\rho v D}{\mu} \qquad (3.1)$$

In Equation 3.1 ρ is the density of the fluid, μ its dynamic viscosity, v the velocity of the fluid and D the characteristic length, which in case of ducts, is usually its diameter.

Hagen-Poiseuille Law establishes the analytical solution of a steady laminar flow of an incompressible fluid through a straight and rigid duct of constant section, subjected to a pressure difference at its ends. The resulting velocity profile is a parabola where the velocity reaches the maximum value on the axis of the duct, reducing to 0 on the walls, as it can be seen in Figure 3.1.

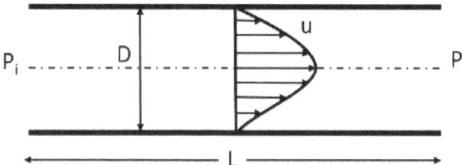

Fig. 3.1 Hagen-Poiseuille velocity profile

The flow rate Q is calculated using Equation 3.2, D is the diameter of the duct, L the length, ΔP the pressure difference between the ends of the duct, μ the dynamic viscosity and Γ is a dimensionless parameter that depends on the geometry (for circular section $\Gamma = \pi/32$).

$$Q = \Gamma \cdot \frac{\Delta P \cdot D^4}{\mu \cdot L} \qquad (3.2)$$

The Hagen-Poiseuille flow introduces numerous simplifications such as Newtonian fluid, laminar flow, steady flow and cylindrical geometry [14]:

- **Newtonian fluid**. Blood is actually a non-Newtonian fluid, but when it is subjected to high velocity gradients ($\partial u/\partial r$) its behavior is more similar to that of a Newtonian fluid, as in the arteries of more than 0.5 mm of diameter.

- **Laminar flow**. To determine if a flow is laminar or turbulent, Reynolds number, previously defined, is used. The typical range of Reynolds numbers in the blood vessels can range from 1 in the small arterioles to approximately 4000 in the aortic artery during the systolic peak [40]. This would be the most unfavorable case, although on average it does not exceed the critical Reynolds for a straight and rigid circular section duct (2300).

  However, it must be said that the blood vessels are neither straight nor rigid and the section is not perfectly circular. For that reason, the critical Reynolds for a blood vessel would be approximately 500 [24].

- **No slippage on the walls**. The layer of blood closest to the arterial wall is firmly attached to it, so this non-slip condition is entirely reasonable.

- **Steady flow**. The blood flow has a pulsating character: accelerations and decelerations appear in the flow, which are not taken into account under the assumption of steady flow.

  Therefore, this approach could only be interesting when it is intended to have an order of magnitude of the average flow with the consequent simplification in the mathematical approach that this entails.

- **Cylindrical geometry**. Arteries can be considered to have roughly circular cross sections, unlike veins, whose shape is more closely to an ellipse.

3.2 Dimensionless numbers

- **Rigid walls**. Arterial walls are flexible and deform with pressure changes throughout the cardiac cycle, whereby the interaction between flow and wall deformation has a not inconsiderable effect.

- **Flow developed**. In the bifurcations the velocity profile is not parabolic until it exceeds the detachment zone in the entrance region and it can be considered developed flow. The length of the detachment zone depends on the Reynolds number.

These assumptions deviate from the actual blood flow. However, in certain cases it can be considered as a good first approximation of the blood flow.

Blood flow is considered in most cases as laminar flow. However, it is pulsatile and under certain conditions and in small time intervals the flow can be dominated by inertial forces [14].

So another dimensionless parameter, the **Womersley number**, is used to characterize an unsteady flow. The velocity profile of a pulsating flow depends on the size of the duct D, the angular frequency of the pulse ω and the density ρ and viscosity μ of the fluid. This is reflected in the Womersley dimensionless parameter, Wo, which expresses the importance of unsteady inertial forces versus viscous forces.

$$Wo = \frac{D}{2} \cdot \sqrt{\frac{\omega \cdot \rho}{\mu}} \qquad (3.3)$$

For low Womersley parameter values ($Wo < 1$), as in narrow vessels and with low frequency values, the viscous stresses will dominate and we will have a quasi-stationary parabolic velocity profile governed by Poiseuille's Law. For higher values ($1 < Wo < 3$) the instantaneous velocity profile lags behind the instantaneous pressure gradient. If the values are already very high ($Wo > 4$), inertia dominates the viscous effects and the velocity profile becomes practically flat and the flow has a marked unsteady character [69].

Figure 3.2 shows the evolution of the velocity profile for different instants of time in a cycle with a sinusoidal pressure gradient. It is observed that at certain moments of the cycle, if the Womersley number is high, the velocity at the points near the wall differs from the velocities in the center of the section, where the velocity profile is practically flat.

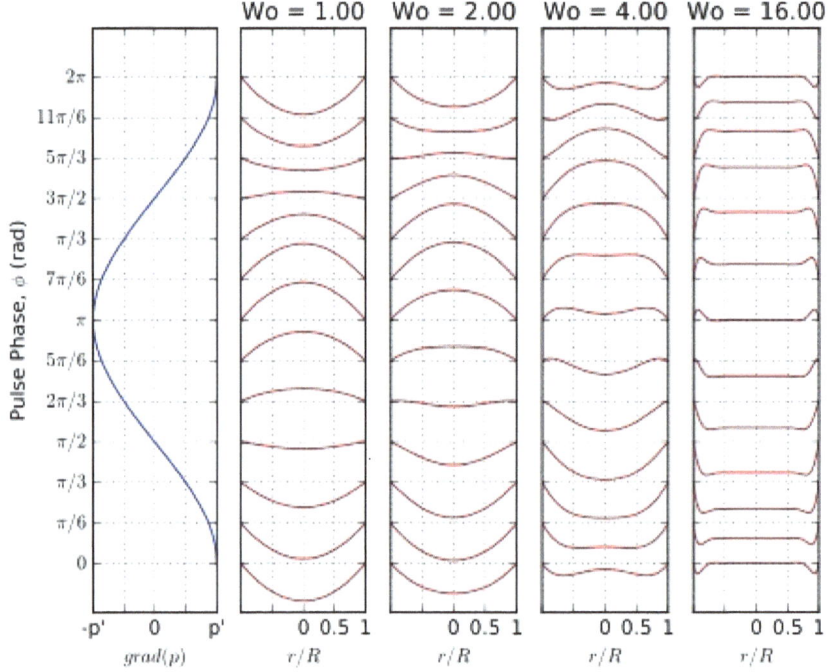

Fig. 3.2 Theoretical velocity profile in a cycle for different Womersley numbers[1]

---
[1]Adapted from: https://wikivisually.com/wiki/Pulsatile_flow

3.3 Fluid-mechanical description of the flow in the Left Atrial Appendage

In this section, a fluid dynamic characterization of the flow in the LAA is performed to define the boundary conditions to be reproduced in the numerical models. It is essential to reproduce the flow pattern, Reynolds and Womersley numbers in the Left Atrial and LAA.

3.3.1 Flow pattern

The location and orientation of the inlets of the four pulmonary veins in the left atrium may vary depending on the patient. Several studies such as that of Dahl et al. [17], in which they obtained geometries with MRI or in the one by Olivares et al. [50], who obtained them through 3D Rotational Angiography, agreed to use for their studies a geometry similar to that shown in the simplified model in Figure 3.3.

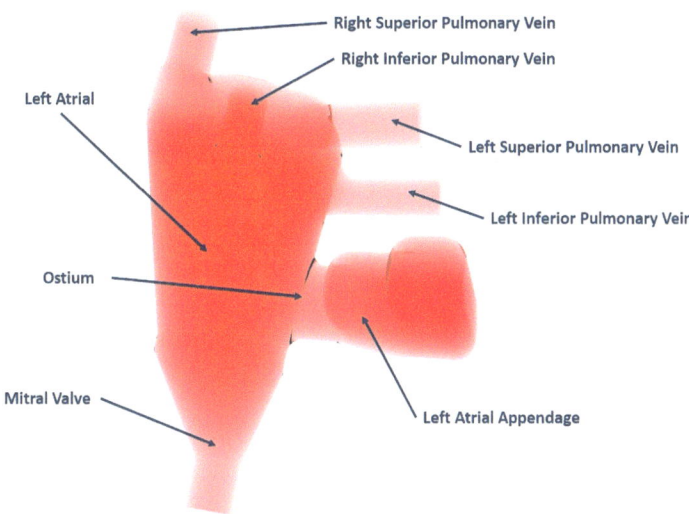

Fig. 3.3 Simplified model of the Left Atrial and Left Atrial Appendage

It can be seen in Figure 3.3 that the inlet of the right pulmonary veins is more aligned and oriented towards the mitral valve, while those of the left veins are made more transversely, as described by Fyrenius et al. [25]. This description of the inflow into the left atrium from the pulmonary veins is also seen in the CFD study performed by Olivares et al. [50].

The flow pattern in the left atrium described in previous sections is similar to that obtained by Vedula et al. [63] using CFD. During diastole the mitral valve is open and the flow from the pulmonary veins is directed towards it to pass into the left ventricle. The transverse entry of the flow from the left pulmonary veins causes the appearance of a vortex (whose axis is parallel to the mitral valve) towards the middle of the diastole period. In contrast, during systole the mitral valve is closed and the generated vortex (also parallel to the mitral valve) is of greater magnitude than in diastole.

3.3.2 Boundary conditions

One of the fundamental parts of numerical models validation (*in vitro* and *in vivo*) is the choice of adequate boundary conditions. Apart from that, it is necessary to know the most relevant techniques to study the flow in the study region in order to compare with the flow obtained with CFD simulations.

In order to perform an adequate validation of the CFD model, it is not enough to only make a qualitative or quantitative comparison, but it is also necessary to establish a methodology for calculating errors such as it is shown in the scheme in Figure 3.4.

3.3 Fluid-mechanical description of the flow in the LAA 47

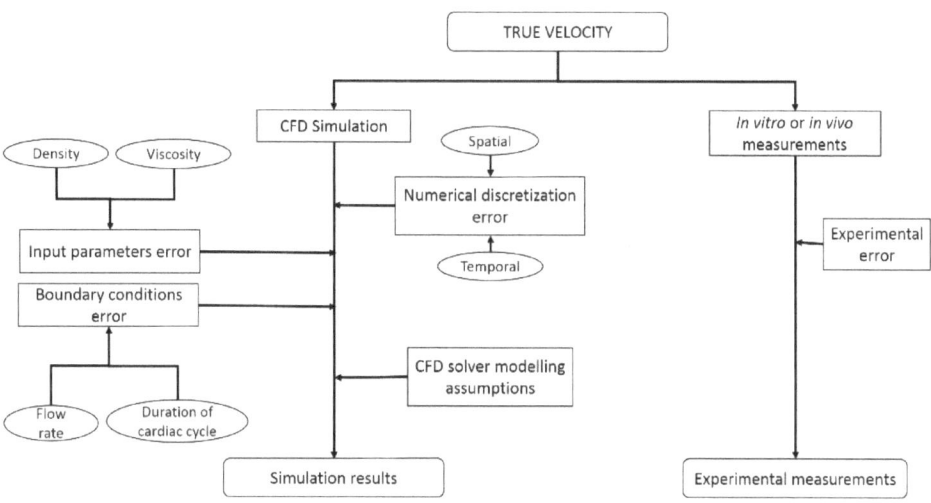

Fig. 3.4 Estimation of errors in CFD models and in experimental measurements

Next, boundary conditions relative to the bibliography will be detailed. There is great variability in the data found, especially in terms of dimensions as they vary during the cardiac cycle. The aim is to reproduce those flow conditions in simulations with Reynolds and Womersley numbers that are close to reality.

3.3.2.1 Pulmonary veins

Table 3.1 shows the dimensions of the pulmonary veins obtained with MRI for the study by Dahl et al. [17]. It can be seen that there is a larger and a smaller diameter since the section of the pulmonary veins is not completely circular, but elliptical. Furthermore, the sections of the right pulmonary veins are slightly larger than the left ones.

Fernández-Pérez et al. [23] obtained from MRI the velocity curve in a pulmonary vein for a healthy patient. In systole the peak velocity is approximately 0.18 m/s while the peak velocity reached in diastole is 0.24 m/s.

Table 3.1 Pulmonary veins sections obtained with MRI [17]

	LSPV	LIPV	RSPV	RIPV
Minor axis (*mm*)	11.9	10.6	12.1	16.1
Major axis (*mm*)	15.4	15.8	17.0	16.1
Area (*mm²*)	113.8	131.2	156.4	203.1

Koizumi et al. [38] took data about the inflow of a pulmonary vein using MRI for their computational study, differentiating between a healthy patient and patients with atrial fibrillation. For healthy patients, it can be seen that the maximum flow rates are between 30-40 mL/s although there are several oscillations in the flow curve.

Lantz et al. [41] indicate that as a first approximation it can be assumed that 25% of the total flow entering the left atrium from the pulmonary veins circulates through each pulmonary vein, but according to measurements obtained in vivo MRI may not always be the case as it depends on each patient. They also carried out a CFD case to study the effect of the variation in the flow rates of the pulmonary veins. They concluded that the flow in the left atrium is strongly influenced by these flow variations in the pulmonary veins. Instead, the mitral valve regulates flow and minimizes these effects on the left ventricle.

3.3.2.2 Mitral valve

In diastole, just after the mitral valve opens, the left ventricle fills rapidly and the velocity peak is reached through the mitral valve, reaching up to 0.5 m/s, although the most usual value is 0.33 m/s [23]. The maximum flow rate through the mitral valve is approximately 150 mL/s [38]. The last smaller peak coincides with atrial contraction, causing the reduced filling stage of the ventricle.

3.3 Fluid-mechanical description of the flow in the LAA

The opening and closing time of the mitral valve is less than 5% of the duration of the cardiac cycle so it can be considered practically instantaneous because it usually does not exceed 50 ms [15].

In contrast, the process of closing the mitral valve is more complex than that of opening. After rapid filling of the left ventricle, the mitral valve is partially closed and the flow decelerates. Once the reduced filling produced by the atrial contraction is finished, the mitral valve closes completely [71].

The mitral annulus is elliptical and varies in shape and size during the cardiac cycle [51]. In the bibliography there are very different values for its section, but during diastole its shape is more circular and can be approximated by a circle with a diameter of 24 mm [38].

The Reynolds number referred to the diameter of the mean mitral annulus during the peak of diastole is 2420 while the Womersley number referred to the diameter of the mitral annulus and the duration of the cardiac cycle is 19 [63].

3.3.2.3 Left Atrial Appendage

The diameter of the **Ostium** varies considerably from one patient to another (from 10 to 40 mm), as can be extracted from the study carried out by Ernst et al. [21].

The blood flow rates in the LAA originate mainly from the volume variation (contraction and dilation) that this appendage experiences during the cardiac cycle. The LAA dilates during ventricular systole as the mitral valve is closed and fluid recirculation to it occurs. Later, during ventricular diastole, a volume contraction occurs to discharge the fluid stored during the previous stage into the left ventricle through the mitral valve, now open. This decrease in volume is drastic during atrial contraction.

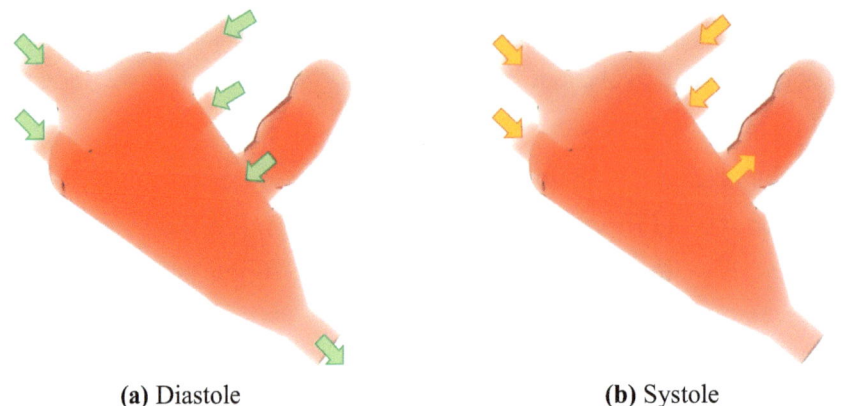

(a) Diastole (b) Systole

Fig. 3.5 Flows in a simplified Left Atrial and Left Atrial Appendage model

The volume variation experienced by the LAA is the same during systole and during diastole, but since these two stages have different durations, the flow rates will not be the same and will be calculated using Equation 3.4.

$$\Delta V_{LAA} = Q_{LAA(systole)} \cdot t_{systole} = Q_{LAA(diastole)} \cdot t_{diastole} \qquad (3.4)$$

Taking into account the approximate duration of diastole (600 ms) and systole (400 ms), the flow rate in the LAA during systole will be 1.5 times the flow rate in the LAA during diastole.

$$\frac{Q_{LAA(systole)}}{Q_{LAA(diastole)}} \approx 1.5 \qquad (3.5)$$

The physiological conditions most prone to thrombus formation in the LAA occur in patients with atrial fibrillation in whom the LAA has lost its ability to contract [50], since there is hardly any volume variation in the LAA (<5 mL) during the cardiac cycle.

The left atrium also presents a reduction in the contraction capacity when the patient has atrial fibrillation. One way to estimate this contraction capacity is using the atrial ejection fraction, EF_{LA}, defined as:

$$EF_{LA} = \frac{V_{LA(max)} - V_{LA(min)}}{V_{LA(max)}} \qquad (3.6)$$

The higher EF_{LA} the more contraction capacity the atrium has. In a person with sinus rhythm, the ejection fraction of the atrium is around 45.4% ± 13.9%, while if he suffers from atrial fibrillation, it is 26.3% ± 10.4% [32].

Although data about flows and dimensions related to the left atrium and left atrial appendage have been collected, the numerical values are indicative due to the great variability in terms of morphology and flow rates in the heart.

3.4 State of the art about the flow in the Left Atrial Appendage

There is a clear interest in the experimental and computational study of the LAA and left atrium. However, there are few publications that deal with the problem from the perspective of fluid mechanics. Vedula et al. [63] conducted studies on patient-specific geometries, highlighting the role of vortex formation and its influence on the left atrium and left atrial appendage.

Otani et al. [52] identified the vortices formed in the left atrium and LAA using the Q criterion in patient-specific geometries and made a basic fluid-dynamic study. Olivares et al. [50] dealt with the problem analyzing different types of basic LAA geometry already discussed and introduces them into their computational model, with the aim of relating vortical structures with the risk of thrombosis.

They also used the Q criterion for vortex identification to relate flow to thrombosis risk. This criterion has a fairly low efficiency detecting vortices in non-steady flows [30].

García-Isla et al. [28] carried out a study in which they analyzed different basic LAA geometries through a CFD model without volume variation to study the risk of thrombosis in this area, establishing as a contour condition the velocity in a pulmonary vein.

The average velocities obtained in the Ostium for the average dimensions of the LAA morphologies are higher than those that would correspond to the volume variations experienced in the LAA because boundary conditions of both Olivares et al. [50] as de García-Isla et al. [28] did not take into account the reverse flow in the pulmonary veins at the end of diastole, unlike Fyrenius et al. [25] or Fernández-Pérez et al. [23].

Bosi et al. [10] also conducted a CFD study of a rigid model with the aim of comparing the results that would be obtained in healthy patients with those who have atrial fibrillation. They established the condition of velocity contour in the mitral valve, differentiating the case of sinus rhythm with the two velocity peaks in diastole and the case of atrial fibrillation, in which the last peak produced by atrial contraction has disappeared due to the reduced contraction capacity of the patient. They obtained the velocities in the LAA as a function of the distance to the Ostium for the four basic types of geometry. They also spatially integrated these velocities into the LAA volume and normalized it with respect to said volume. They concluded that the LAA velocities were lower in case of atrial fibrillation, with Chicken wing and Cauliflower morphologies presenting a greater thromboembolic risk.

In most of the investigations carried out, the study of the LAA is approached taking into account the morphological classification presented by Yan et al. [67] with the quantitative limits of Kimura et al. [36]: Cactus, ChickenWing, WindSock and CauliFlower.

According to the study carried out by Di Biase et al. [8] the Cauliflower morphology is the one with the highest thromboembolic risk. However, this morphology classification of the LAA is not too clear and may depend on the perspective from which the LAA is observed [5].

3.4 State of the art about the flow in the Left Atrial Appendage

Kosiuk et al. [39] studied the risk of thrombosis evaluating platelet activation in patients with atrial fibrillation. They did not find a clear dependence on the morphology of the LAA, although they did obtain higher activation states (greater thromboembolic risk) if the LAA volume was greater.

Masci et al. [46] carried out a CFD study of a model with volume variation of the left atrium and LAA from MDCT images. To simulate the alteration of the heart rate in case of atrial fibrillation, they introduced a random displacement (≈ 0.01 mm) of the nodes, in addition to eliminating the A wave of the flow through the mitral valve.

Regarding the study of occlusion devices for the LAA, Aguado et al. [1] carried out a CFD study to optimize the choice of the occluder device, as well as its size and settlement area. They simulated the two most widely used types of occluder devices, the Amplatzer Amulet and the Watchman, in a rigid left atrial and LAA model.

Jia et al. [34] also studied with CFD the effect of the introduction of an occluder device in the LAA. They compared the flow pattern, velocities, and vorticity obtained in a rigid model with LAA and without LAA to observe the effect of the appendage closure. In case of LAA occlusion, vortices of the left atrium reduce their duration and intensity, indicating that the associated risk of thrombosis is lower.

There is a clear need for knowledge generation in this area. The limitations of existing studies are many because all studies assume that the flow created in the left atrium and LAA is laminar. Nowadays, it is not possible to say with certainty whether the flow is laminar or not throughout the cardiac cycle or during arrhythmia due to the lack of experimental and numerical results. In addition, there is also little information about boundary conditions of velocities or pressures, essential for consistent validation.

References

[1] Aguado, A. M., Olivares, A. L., Yagüe, C., Silva, E., Nuñez-García, M., Fernandez-Quilez, Á., Mill, J., Genua, I., Arzamendi, D., Potter, T. D., Freixa, X., and Camara, O. (2019). In silico optimization of left atrial appendage occluder implantation using interactive and modeling tools. *Frontiers in Physiology*, 10.

[2] Al-Saady, N. M., Obel, O. A., and Camm, A. J. (1999). Left atrial appendage: structure, function, and role in thromboembolism. *Heart*, 82(5):547–554.

[3] Anselmino, M., Matta, M., D'Ascenzo, F., Bunch, T. J., Schilling, R. J., Hunter, R. J., Pappone, C., Neumann, T., Noelker, G., Fiala, M., Bertaglia, E., Frontera, A., Duncan, E., Nalliah, C., Jais, P., Weerasooriya, R., Kalman, J. M., and Gaita, F. (2014). Catheter ablation of atrial fibrillation in patients with left ventricular systolic dysfunction. *Circulation: Arrhythmia and Electrophysiology*, 7(6):1011–1018.

[4] Atienza, F. and Moya, Á. (2016). Tratamiento no farmacológico de la fibrilación auricular. ablación, cardioversión eléctrica, marcapasos y cierre de la orejuela. *Revista Española de Cardiología Suplementos*, 16:40–46.

[5] Beigel, R., Wunderlich, N. C., Ho, S. Y., Arsanjani, R., and Siegel, R. J. (2014). The left atrial appendage: Anatomy, function, and noninvasive evaluation. *JACC: Cardiovascular Imaging*, 7(12):1251 – 1265.

[6] Bermejo, J., Martínez-Legazpi, P., and del Álamo, J. C. (2015). The clinical assessment of intraventricular flows. *Annual Review of Fluid Mechanics*, 47(1):315–342.

[7] Biase, L. D., Burkhardt, J. D., Mohanty, P., Sanchez, J., Mohanty, S., Horton, R., Gallinghouse, G. J., Bailey, S. M., Zagrodzky, J. D., Santangeli,

P., Hao, S., Hongo, R., Beheiry, S., Themistoclakis, S., Bonso, A., Rossillo, A., Corrado, A., Raviele, A., Al-Ahmad, A., Wang, P., Cummings, J. E., Schweikert, R. A., Pelargonio, G., Russo, A. D., Casella, M., Santarelli, P., Lewis, W. R., and Natale, A. (2010). Left atrial appendage. *Circulation*, 122(2):109–118.

[8] Biase, L. D., Santangeli, P., Anselmino, M., Mohanty, P., Salvetti, I., Gili, S., Horton, R., Sanchez, J. E., Bai, R., Mohanty, S., Pump, A., Brantes, M. C., Gallinghouse, G. J., Burkhardt, J. D., Cesarani, F., Scaglione, M., Natale, A., and Gaita, F. (2012). Does the left atrial appendage morphology correlate with the risk of stroke in patients with atrial fibrillation?: Results from a multicenter study. *Journal of the American College of Cardiology*, 60(6):531 – 538.

[9] Blackshear, J. L. and Odell, J. A. (1996). Appendage obliteration to reduce stroke in cardiac surgical patients with atrial fibrillation. *The Annals of Thoracic Surgery*, 61(2):755–759.

[10] Bosi, G. M., Cook, A., Rai, R., Menezes, L. J., Schievano, S., Torii, R., and Burriesci, G. (2018). Computational fluid dynamic analysis of the left atrial appendage to predict thrombosis risk. *Frontiers in Cardiovascular Medicine*, 5.

[11] Buchmann, N. A., Yamamoto, M., Jermy, M., and David, T. (2010). Particle image velocimetry (PIV) and computational fluid dynamics (CFD) modelling of carotid artery haemodynamics under steady flow: A validation study. *Journal of Biomechanical Science and Engineering*, 5(4):421– 436.

[12] Buckmaster and Vicol (2019). Nonuniqueness of weak solutions to the navier-stokes equation. *Annals of Mathematics*, 189(1):101.

[13] Burrell, L. D., Horne, B. D., Anderson, J. L., Muhlestein, J. B., and Whisenant, B. K. (2013). Usefulness of left atrial appendage volume as a predictor of embolic stroke in patients with atrial fibrillation. *The American Journal of Cardiology*, 112(8):1148–1152.

[14] Chandran, K. B., Rittgers, S. E., and Yoganathan, A. P. (2012). *Biofluid Mechanics: The Human Circulation, Second Edition*. CRC Press.

[15] Chnafa, C., Mendez, S., and Nicoud, F. (2014). Image-based large-eddy simulation in a realistic left heart. *Computers & Fluids*, 94:173–187.

References

[16] Chung, B. and Cebral, J. R. (2014). CFD for evaluation and treatment planning of aneurysms: Review of proposed clinical uses and their challenges. *Annals of Biomedical Engineering*, 43(1):122–138.

[17] Dahl, S. K., Thomassen, E., Hellevik, L. R., and Skallerud, B. (2012). Impact of pulmonary venous locations on the intra-atrial flow and the mitral valve plane velocity profile. *Cardiovascular Engineering and Technology*, 3(3):269–281.

[18] Davis, R. C., Hobbs, F. D. R., Kenkre, J. E., Roalfe, A. K., Iles, R., Lip, G. Y. H., and Davies, M. K. (2012). Prevalence of atrial fibrillation in the general population and in high-risk groups: the ECHOES study. *Europace*, 14(11):1553–1559.

[19] Dentamaro, I., Vestito, D., Michelotto, E., Santis, D. D., Ostuni, V., Cadeddu, C., and Colonna, P. (2016). Evaluation of left atrial appendage function and thrombi in patients with atrial fibrillation: from transthoracic to real time 3d transesophageal echocardiography. *The International Journal of Cardiovascular Imaging*, 33(4):491–498.

[20] Desimone, C. V. and Asirvatham, S. J. (2014). ICE imaging of the left atrial appendage. *Journal of Cardiovascular Electrophysiology*, 25(11):1272–1274.

[21] Ernst, G., Stöllberger, C., Abzieher, F., Veit-Dirscherl, W., Bonner, E., Bibus, B., Schneider, B., and Slany, J. (1995). Morphology of the left atrial appendage. *The Anatomical Record*, 242(4):553–561.

[22] Fernández, A. R. and González, A. B. (2016). Técnicas de imagen en el intervencionismo percutáneo estructural: cierre de comunicación interauricular y oclusión de la orejuela izquierda. *Revista Española de Cardiología*, 69(8):766–777.

[23] Fernández-Pérez, G., Duarte, R., de la Calle, M. C., Calatayud, J., and González, J. S. (2012). Analysis of left ventricular diastolic function using magnetic resonance imaging. *Radiología (English Edition)*, 54(4):295–305.

[24] Ferrari, M., Werner, G. S., Bahrmann, P., Richartz, B. M., and Figulla, H. R. (2006). Turbulent flow as a cause for underestimating coronary flow reserve measured by doppler guide wire. *Cardiovascular Ultrasound*, 4(1).

[25] Fyrenius, A. (2001). Three dimensional flow in the human left atrium. *Heart*, 86(4):448–455.

[26] Gan, C. H. G., Bhat, A., Davis, L., and Denniss, A. R. (2014). Percutaneous transcatheter left atrial appendage closure devices: Role in the long-term management of atrial fibrillation. *Heart, Lung and Circulation*, 23(5):407–413.

[27] García-Fernández, M. A., Torrecilla, E. G., Román, D. S., Azevedo, J., Bueno, H., Moreno, M., and Delcán, J. L. (1992). Left atrial appendage doppler flow patterns: Implications on thrombus formation. *American Heart Journal*, 124(4):955–961.

[28] García-Isla, G., Olivares, A. L., Silva, E., Nuñez-Garcia, M., Butakoff, C., Sanchez-Quintana, D., Morales, H. G., Freixa, X., Noailly, J., Potter, T. D., and Camara, O. (2018). Sensitivity analysis of geometrical parameters to study haemodynamics and thrombus formation in the left atrial appendage. *International Journal for Numerical Methods in Biomedical Engineering*, 34(8):e3100.

[29] Hall, J. E. (2010). *Guyton and Hall Textbook of Medical Physiology, 12e*. Saunders.

[30] Haller, G. (2015). Lagrangian coherent structures. *Annual Review of Fluid Mechanics*, 47(1):137–162.

[31] Holmes, J. W. and Wagenseil, J. E. (2016). Special issue: Spotlight on the future of cardiovascular engineering: Frontiers and challenges in cardiovascular biomechanics. *Journal of Biomechanical Engineering*, 138(11):110301.

[32] Hwang, S. H., Roh, S. Y., Shim, J., il Choi, J., Kim, Y.-H., and Oh, Y.-W. (2017). Atrial fibrillation: Relationship between left atrial pressure and left atrial appendage emptying determined with velocity-encoded cardiac MR imaging. *Radiology*, 284(2):381–389.

[33] Itatani, K., Miyazaki, S., Furusawa, T., Numata, S., Yamazaki, S., Morimoto, K., Makino, R., Morichi, H., Nishino, T., and Yaku, H. (2017). New imaging tools in cardiovascular medicine: computational fluid dynamics and 4d flow MRI. *General Thoracic and Cardiovascular Surgery*, 65(11):611–621.

[34] Jia, D., Jeon, B., Park, H.-B., Chang, H.-J., and Zhang, L. T. (2019). Image-based flow simulations of pre- and post-left atrial appendage closure in the left atrium. *Cardiovascular Engineering and Technology*, 10(2):225–241.

[35] Kanderian, A. S., Gillinov, A. M., Pettersson, G. B., Blackstone, E., and Klein, A. L. (2008). Success of surgical left atrial appendage closure. *Journal of the American College of Cardiology*, 52(11):924–929.

[36] Kimura, T., Takatsuki, S., Inagawa, K., Katsumata, Y., Nishiyama, T., Nishiyama, N., Fukumoto, K., Aizawa, Y., Tanimoto, Y., Tanimoto, K., Jinzaki, M., and Fukuda, K. (2013). Anatomical characteristics of the left atrial appendage in cardiogenic stroke with low CHADS2 scores. *Heart Rhythm*, 10(6):921–925.

[37] Klabunde, R. E. (2011). *Cardiovascular Physiology Concepts*. Lippincott Williams&Wilki.

[38] Koizumi, R., Funamoto, K., Hayase, T., Kanke, Y., Shibata, M., Shiraishi, Y., and Yambe, T. (2015). Numerical analysis of hemodynamic changes in the left atrium due to atrial fibrillation. *Journal of Biomechanics*, 48(3):472 – 478.

[39] Kosiuk, J., Uhe, T., Stegmann, C., Ueberham, L., Bertagnolli, L., Dagres, N., Dinov, B., Müssigbrodt, A., Richter, S., Paetsch, I., Jahnke, C., Hilbert, S., Sommer, P., Hindricks, G., and Bollmann, A. (2019). Morphological determinators of platelet activation status in patients with atrial fibrillation. *International Journal of Cardiology*, 279:90–95.

[40] Ku, D. N. (1997). Blood Flow in Arteries. *Annual Review of Fluid Mechanics*, 29(1):399–434.

[41] Lantz, J., Gupta, V., Henriksson, L., Karlsson, M., Persson, A., Carlhäll, C.-J., and Ebbers, T. (2018). Impact of pulmonary venous inflow on cardiac flow simulations: Comparison with in vivo 4d flow MRI. *Annals of Biomedical Engineering*, 47(2):413–424.

[42] López-Mínguez, J. R., González-Fernández, R., Fernández-Vegas, C., Millán-Nuñez, V., Fuentes-Cañamero, M. E., Nogales-Asensio, J. M., Doncel-Vecino, J., Elduayen-Gragera, J., Ho, S. Y., and Sánchez-Quintana, D. (2014). Anatomical classification of left atrial appendages in specimens applicable to CT imaging techniques for implantation of amplatzer cardiac plug. *Journal of Cardiovascular Electrophysiology*, 25(9):976–984.

[43] Marek, D., Vindis, D., and Kocianova, E. (2013). Real time 3-dimensional transesophageal echocardiography is more specific than 2-dimensional TEE in the assessment of left atrial appendage thrombosis. *Biomedical Papers*, 157(1):22–26.

[44] Markl, M., Lee, D. C., Carr, M. L., Foucar, C., Ng, J., Schnell, S., Carr, J. C., and Goldberger, J. J. (2015). Assessment of left atrial and left atrial appendage flow and stasis in atrial fibrillation. *Journal of Cardiovascular Magnetic Resonance*, 17(Suppl 1):M3.

[45] Markl, M., Lee, D. C., Furiasse, N., Carr, M., Foucar, C., Ng, J., Carr, J., and Goldberger, J. J. (2016). Left atrial and left atrial appendage 4d blood flow dynamics in atrial fibrillation. *Circulation: Cardiovascular Imaging*, 9(9).

[46] Masci, A., Alessandrini, M., Forti, D., Menghini, F., Dedé, L., Tommasi, C., Quarteroni, A., and Corsi, C. (2017). A patient-specific computational fluid dynamics model of the left atrium in atrial fibrillation: Development and initial evaluation. In *Functional Imaging and Modelling of the Heart*, pages 392–400. Springer International Publishing.

[47] Morillo, C. A., Banerjee, A., Perel, P., Wood, D. A., and Jouven, X. P. (2017). Atrial fibrillation: the current epidemic. In *Journal of geriatric cardiology : JGC*.

[48] Nakajima, H., Seo, Y., Ishizu, T., Yamamoto, M., Machino, T., Harimura, Y., Kawamura, R., Sekiguchi, Y., Tada, H., and Aonuma, K. (2010). Analysis of the left atrial appendage by three-dimensional transesophageal echocardiography. *The American Journal of Cardiology*, 106(6):885–892.

[49] Nucifora, G., Faletra, F. F., Regoli, F., Pasotti, E., Pedrazzini, G., Moccetti, T., and Auricchio, A. (2011). Evaluation of the left atrial appendage with real-time 3-dimensional transesophageal echocardiography. *Circulation: Cardiovascular Imaging*, 4(5):514–523.

[50] Olivares, A. L., Silva, E., Nuñez-Garcia, M., Butakoff, C., Sánchez-Quintana, D., Freixa, X., Noailly, J., de Potter, T., and Camara, O. (2017). In silico analysis of haemodynamics in patient-specific left atria with different appendage morphologies. In Pop, M. and Wright, G. A., editors, *Functional Imaging and Modelling of the Heart*, pages 412–420, Cham. Springer International Publishing.

[51] Ormiston, J. A., Shah, P. M., Tei, C., and Wong, M. (1981). Size and motion of the mitral valve annulus in man. i. a two-dimensional echocardiographic method and findings in normal subjects. *Circulation*, 64(1):113–120.

[52] Otani, T., Al-Issa, A., Pourmorteza, A., McVeigh, E. R., Wada, S., and Ashikaga, H. (2016). A computational framework for personalized blood flow analysis in the human left atrium. *Annals of Biomedical Engineering*, 44(11):3284–3294.

[53] Otto, C. M., Schwaegler, R. G., and Freeman, R. V. (2011). *Echocardiography Review Guide: Companion to the Textbook of Clinical Echocardiography: Expert Consult: Online and Print*. Saunders.

[54] Paolinelli, G. P. (2013). Principios físicos e indicaciones clínicas del ultrasonido doppler. *Revista Médica Clínica Las Condes*, 24(1):139 – 148. Tema central: Radiología al día.

[55] Prinz, C., Faludi, R., Walker, A., Amzulescu, M., Gao, H., Uejima, T., Fraser, A. G., and Voigt, J.-U. (2012). Can echocardiographic particle image velocimetry correctly detect motion patterns as they occur in blood inside heart chambers? a validation study using moving phantoms. *Cardiovascular Ultrasound*, 10(1).

[56] Rayz, V. L., Boussel, L., Acevedo-Bolton, G., Martin, A. J., Young, W. L., Lawton, M. T., Higashida, R., and Saloner, D. (2008). Numerical simulations of flow in cerebral aneurysms: Comparison of CFD results and in vivo MRI measurements. *Journal of Biomechanical Engineering*, 130(5):051011.

[57] Scherr, D., Dalal, D., Chilukuri, K., Dong, J., Spragg, D., Henrikson, C. A., Nazarian, S., Cheng, A., Berger, R. D., Abraham, T. P., Calkins, H., and Marine, J. E. (2009). Incidence and predictors of left atrial thrombus prior to catheter ablation of atrial fibrillation. *Journal of Cardiovascular Electrophysiology*, 20(4):379–384.

[58] Soldevila, J. G., Ruíz, M. D. M., Robert, I. D., Tornos, P., and Martínez-Rubio, A. (2013). Evaluación de riesgo tromboembólico y hemorrágico de los pacientes con fibrilación auricular. *Revista Española de Cardiología Suplementos*, 13:9–13.

[59] Stoddard, M. F., Dawkins, P. R., Prince, C. R., and Ammash, N. M. (1995). Left atrial appendage thrombus is not uncommon in patients with

acute atrial fibrillation and a recent embolic event: A transesophageal echocardiographics tudy. *Journal of the American College of Cardiology*, 25(2):452–459.

[60] Tabata, T., Oki, T., Fukuda, N., Iuchi, A., Manabe, K., Kageji, Y., Sasaki, M., Yamada, H., and Ito, S. (1996). Influence of aging on left atrial appendage flow velocity patterns in normal subjects. *Journal of the American Society of Echocardiography*, 9(3):274–280.

[61] Thondapu, V., Bourantas, C. V., Foin, N., Jang, I.-K., Serruys, P. W., and Barlis, P. (2016). Biomechanical stress in coronary atherosclerosis: emerging insights from computational modelling. *European Heart Journal*, page ehv689.

[62] van de Vosse, F. N. and Stergiopulos, N. (2011). Pulse wave propagation in the arterial tree. *Annual Review of Fluid Mechanics*, 43(1):467–499.

[63] Vedula, V., George, R., Younes, L., and Mittal, R. (2015). Hemodynamics in the left atrium and its effect on ventricular flow patterns. *Journal of Biomechanical Engineering*.

[64] Veinot, J. P., Harrity, P. J., Gentile, F., Khandheria, B. K., Bailey, K. R., Eickholt, J. T., Seward, J. B., Tajik, A. J., and Edwards, W. D. (1997). Anatomy of the normal left atrial appendage. *Circulation*, 96(9):3112–3115.

[65] Vigna, C., Russo, A., Rito, V. D., Perna, G., Villella, A., Testa, M., Sollazzo, V., Fanelli, R., and Loperfido, F. (1992). Frequency of left atrial thrombi by transesophageal echocardiography in idiopathic and in ischemic dilated cardiomyopathy. *The American Journal of Cardiology*, 70(18):1500–1501.

[66] Vlachopoulos, C., O'Rourke, M., and Nichols, W. W. (2011). *McDonald's Blood Flow in Arteries, Sixth Edition: Theoretical, Experimental and Clinical Principles*. HODDER & STROUGHTON.

[67] Wang, Y., Biase, L. D., Horton, R. P., Nguyen, T., Morhanty, P., and Natale, A. (2010). Left atrial appendage studied by computed tomography to help planning for appendage closure device placement. *Journal of Cardiovascular Electrophysiology*, 21(9):973–982.

[68] Yamamoto, M., Seo, Y., Kawamatsu, N., Sato, K., Sugano, A., Machino-Ohtsuka, T., Kawamura, R., Nakajima, H., Igarashi, M., Sekiguchi, Y.,

Ishizu, T., and Aonuma, K. (2014). Complex left atrial appendage morphology and left atrial appendage thrombus formation in patients with atrial fibrillation. *Circulation: Cardiovascular Imaging*, 7(2):337–343.

[69] Yazdi, S. G., Geoghegan, P. H., Docherty, P. D., Jermy, M., and Khanafer, A. (2018). A review of arterial phantom fabrication methods for flow measurement using piv techniques. *Annals of Biomedical Engineering*, 46(11):1697–1721.

[70] Yin, W. and Frame, M. D. (2011). *Biofluid Mechanics: An Introduction to Fluid Mechanics, Macrocirculation, and Microcirculation (Biomedical Engineering)*. Academic Press.

[71] Yoganathan, A. P., He, Z., and Jones, S. C. (2004). Fluid mechanics of heart valves. *Annual Review of Biomedical Engineering*, 6(1):331–362.